Fatty Liver Diet

Cookbook

For Seniors 2024

Energizing Recipes for Optimal Liver Function Detoxification & a Long Healthy Life

Dr. Olivia Tastewell

The recipes and information in this book are based on the author's personal experience and research. They are not intended to replace the advice of your doctor or health care provider. Please consult your doctor before making any changes to your diet or lifestyle. The author and publisher are not responsible for any adverse effects or consequences resulting from the use of any of the recipes or information in this book.

The author hopes that this book will inspire you to enjoy cooking and eating healthy and delicious food. She welcomes your feedback and suggestions and invites you to share your recipes and stories with her. Thank you for choosing this book and supporting the author's work.

Dr Olivia Tastewell
Author Fatty Liver Air Fryer Cookbook
Email: droliviatastewell@gmail.com

TABLE OF CONTENT

INTRODUCTION..5

Breakfast Recipes...9

Greek Yogurt with Berries and Chia Seeds.......9

Scrambled Eggs with Spinach and Tomatoes. 10

Oatmeal with Banana and Nuts......................11

Avocado Toast with Smoked Salmon..............12

Smoothie with Spinach, Banana, and Almond Milk..13

Lunch Recipes... 15

Tuna Salad with Whole Wheat Crackers........ 15

Lentil Soup with Whole Wheat Bread............. 16

Chicken Caesar Salad with Light Dressing..... 17

Black Bean and Corn Salad with Avocado......18

Leftover Grilled Chicken or Fish with Roasted Vegetables.. 19

Dinner Recipes...21

Air-Fried Salmon with Roasted Broccoli..........21

Chicken Stir-Fry with Brown Rice and Vegetables... 23

Baked Sweet Potato with Black Beans and Salsa.. 25

Shrimp Scampi over Zoodles........................27

One-Pan Chicken with Roasted Vegetables... 29

Snacks... 31

Apple Slices with Almond Butter.................... 31

Edamame Pods..32

Carrot Sticks with Hummus............................33

Greek Yogurt with Berries.............................. 34

Air-Fried Chickpeas...35

Drinks...**37**
Green Tea... 37
Water with Lemon or Cucumber..................... 38
Unsweetened Herbal Tea...............................39
Homemade Vegetable Juice.......................... 40
Smoothie with Spinach, Banana, and Water...41
Bonus... 43
Fruit Salad with Chia Seeds...........................43
Hard-boiled Eggs... 44
Cottage Cheese with Fruit..............................45
Air-Fried Tofu Scramble with Vegetables........ 46
Roasted Pumpkin Seeds.................................47
14-Day Meal Plan..**49**
Week 1.. 49
Week 2.. 51
CONCLUSION...**53**

INTRODUCTION

Welcome to the "Fatty Liver Diet Cookbook for Seniors 2024," where we will discuss the crucial subject of fatty liver disease and propose practical answers via tasty and healthy dishes created exclusively for elders. Fatty liver disease, also known as hepatic steatosis, is a condition in which fat accumulates in the liver cells. It is a common and possibly dangerous health condition, particularly among the older population. Sedentary lifestyles, bad eating habits, and underlying health issues are all contributing causes to an increase in the number of seniors dealing with fatty liver disease. Untreated fatty liver disease can lead to serious complications such as liver inflammation (steatohepatitis), permanent liver damage (cirrhosis), and even liver cancer.

As a result, elders must take proactive measures to manage this issue. Our cookbook seeks to provide elders with effective dietary options for managing and perhaps reversing fatty liver disease. We understand the dread and uncertainty that may come with a diagnosis of this ailment, but we are here to offer hope and help. Seniors may take charge of their health and well-being by eating a nutrient-dense, liver-friendly diet. This cookbook has a variety of scrumptious dishes that have been precisely designed to enhance liver health while also pleasing the taste senses. From substantial soups and salads to tasty main courses and indulgent desserts, each meal is intended to be delicious, healthful, and simple to make. Leafy greens, lean meats, healthy fats, and antioxidant-rich fruits and vegetables are among the elements in our meals that have been shown to benefit the liver.

Furthermore, the recipes in this cookbook have been developed with the help of nutritionists and dietitians who specialize in liver health. These culinary inventions are not only delicious, but they are also scientifically shown to improve liver function and general health in seniors. Many people who have adopted these dishes into their diets have reported major changes in their liver function and general quality of life.

So, whether you want to prevent fatty liver disease, manage its symptoms, or just live a healthy lifestyle, the "Fatty Liver Diet Cookbook for Seniors 2024" is your complete guide to culinary wellness. Join us on this path to improved liver health and active life in your older years.

Breakfast Recipes

Greek Yogurt with Berries and Chia Seeds

Serving Size: 1 serving

Ingredients:
- 1/2 cup Greek yogurt
- 1/4 cup mixed berries (such as strawberries, blueberries, raspberries)
- 1 tablespoon chia seeds

Instructions:
1. Transfer the Greek yogurt into a bowl.
2. Top with mixed berries.
3. Sprinkle chia seeds over the berries.
4. Serve immediately and enjoy!

Nutritional Information: (per serving)
Calories: 150 kcal
Protein: 12g, Fat: 5g, Carbohydrates: 15g
Fiber: 7g

Scrambled Eggs with Spinach and Tomatoes

Serving Size: 1 serving

Ingredients:
- 2 large eggs
- 1/2 cup fresh spinach, chopped
- 1/4 cup cherry tomatoes, halved
- Salt and pepper to taste

Instructions:
1. In a bowl, beat the eggs until well combined.
2. Heat a non-stick skillet over medium heat and spray with cooking oil.
3. Add the chopped spinach and cherry tomatoes to the skillet and sauté until the spinach wilts and the tomatoes soften.
4. Pour the beaten eggs into the skillet and scramble until cooked through.
5. To taste, add salt and pepper for seasoning.
6. Transfer to a plate and serve hot.

Nutritional Information: (per serving)
Calories: 220 kcal
Protein: 15g Fat: 14g, Carbohydrates: 8g
Fiber: 3g

Oatmeal with Banana and Nuts

Serving Size: 1 serving

Ingredients:
- 1/2 cup rolled oats
- 1 medium banana, sliced
- 1 tablespoon chopped nuts (such as almonds, walnuts, or pecans)

Instructions:
1. Cook the rolled oats according to package instructions.
2. After cooking, pour the oatmeal into a bowl.
3. Top with sliced banana and chopped nuts.
4. Serve hot and enjoy!

Nutritional Information: (per serving)
Calories: 300 kcal
Protein: 8g, Fat: 10g, Carbohydrates: 45g
Fiber: 7g

Avocado Toast with Smoked Salmon

Serving Size: 1 serving

Ingredients:
- 1 slice whole grain bread, toasted
- 1/2 avocado, mashed
- 2 slices smoked salmon

Instructions:
1. Toast the whole grain bread until golden brown.
2. Spread the mashed avocado evenly over the toasted bread.
3. Top with slices of smoked salmon.
4. Serve immediately and enjoy!

Nutritional Information: (per serving)
Calories: 280 kcal
Protein: 15g, Fat: 18g, Carbohydrates: 20g
Fiber: 7g

Smoothie with Spinach, Banana, and Almond Milk

Serving Size: 1 serving

Ingredients:
- 1 cup fresh spinach leaves
- 1 ripe banana
- 1/2 cup unsweetened almond milk

Instructions:
1. In a blender, combine the fresh spinach leaves, ripe banana, and unsweetened almond milk.
2. Blend until smooth and creamy.
3. Transfer into a glass and serve right away..

Nutritional Information: (per serving)
Calories: 150 kcal
Protein: 4g, Fat: 3g, Carbohydrates: 30g
Fiber: 5g

Lunch Recipes

Tuna Salad with Whole Wheat Crackers

Serving Size: 1 serving

Ingredients:
- 1 can (5 oz) tuna, drained
- 1/4 cup diced celery
- 1 tablespoon light mayonnaise
- Salt and pepper to taste
- Whole wheat crackers for serving

Instructions:
1. In a bowl, combine the drained tuna and diced celery.
2. Add the light mayonnaise and mix well to coat the tuna and celery.
3. To taste, add salt and pepper for seasoning.
4. Serve the tuna salad with whole wheat crackers on the side.
5. Enjoy your protein-rich and satisfying meal!

Nutritional Information: (per serving)
Calories: 200 kcal
Protein: 20g, Fat: 7g, Carbohydrates: 15g
Fiber: 3g

Lentil Soup with Whole Wheat Bread

Serving Size: 1 serving

Ingredients:
- 1/2 cup cooked lentils
- 1 cup low-sodium vegetable broth
- 1/4 cup diced carrots
- 1/4 cup diced onion
- Whole wheat bread for serving

Instructions:
1. In a pot, combine the cooked lentils, low-sodium vegetable broth, diced carrots, and diced onion.
2. Bring the mixture to a boil, then reduce the heat and simmer for 10 minutes until the vegetables are tender.
3. Serve the lentil soup hot with whole wheat bread on the side.
4. Enjoy this hearty and fiber-filled meal!

Nutritional Information: (per serving)
Calories: 250 kcal
Protein: 15g, Fat: 1g, Carbohydrates: 45g
Fiber: 15g

Chicken Caesar Salad with Light Dressing

Serving Size: 1 serving

Ingredients:
- 2 cups chopped romaine lettuce
- 4 oz grilled chicken breast, sliced
- 2 tablespoons light Caesar dressing
- 1 tablespoon grated Parmesan cheese
- Optional: Whole grain croutons

Instructions:
1. In a large bowl, toss the chopped romaine lettuce with the grilled chicken breast slices.
2. Drizzle the light Caesar dressing over the salad and toss to coat evenly.
3. Sprinkle the grated Parmesan cheese on top.
4. Optionally, add whole grain croutons for extra crunch.
5. Serve immediately and enjoy this balanced and satisfying meal!

Nutritional Information: (per serving)
Calories: 300 kcal
Protein: 30g, Fat: 10g, Carbohydrates: 20g
Fiber: 5g

Black Bean and Corn Salad with Avocado

Serving Size: 1 serving

Ingredients:
- 1/2 cup canned black beans, drained and rinsed
- 1/4 cup cooked corn kernels
- 1/4 avocado, diced
- 1 tablespoon lime juice
- Salt and pepper to taste

Instructions:
1. In a bowl, combine the drained black beans, cooked corn kernels, and diced avocado.
2. Drizzle the lime juice over the salad and toss gently to mix.
3. To taste, add salt and pepper for seasoning.
4. Serve immediately and enjoy this plant-based protein and healthy fats meal!

Nutritional Information: (per serving)
Calories: 220 kcal
Protein: 8g, Fat: 10g, Carbohydrates: 30g
Fiber: 10g

Leftover Grilled Chicken or Fish with Roasted Vegetables

Serving Size: 1 serving

Ingredients:
- 4 oz leftover grilled chicken breast or fish fillet
- 1 cup mixed roasted vegetables (such as bell peppers, zucchini, and onions)
- Salt and pepper to taste

Instructions:
1. Reheat the leftover grilled chicken breast or fish fillet if necessary.
2. Serve with mixed roasted vegetables on the side.
3. To taste, add salt and pepper for seasoning.
4. Enjoy this quick and nutritious meal packed with protein and fiber!

Nutritional Information: (per serving)
Calories: 250 kcal
Protein: 30g, Fat: 10g, Carbohydrates: 20g
Fiber: 8g

Dinner Recipes

Air-Fried Salmon with Roasted Broccoli

Serving Size: 1 serving

Ingredients:
- 4 oz salmon fillet
- 1 cup broccoli florets
- 1 tablespoon olive oil
- Salt and pepper to taste
- Lemon wedges for serving

Instructions:
1. Set the air fryer to 200°C or 400°F.
2. Season the salmon fillet with salt, pepper, and a drizzle of olive oil.
3. Place the seasoned salmon fillet in the air fryer basket and cook for 10-12 minutes, or until cooked through and crispy on the outside.
4. Meanwhile, toss the broccoli florets with olive oil, salt, and pepper.
5. Transfer the seasoned broccoli florets to a baking sheet and roast in the oven at 400°F (200°C) for 15-20 minutes, or until tender and slightly charred.
6. Serve the air-fried salmon with roasted broccoli and lemon wedges on the side.

7. Enjoy this easy and omega-3 rich dinner!

Nutritional Information: (per serving)
Calories: 300 kcal
Protein: 25g, Fat: 15g, Carbohydrates: 10g
Fiber: 5g

Chicken Stir-Fry with Brown Rice and Vegetables

Serving Size: 1 serving

Ingredients:
- 4 oz cooked chicken breast, sliced
- 1 cup cooked brown rice
- 1 cup mixed stir-fry vegetables (such as bell peppers, carrots, and snap peas)
- 2 tablespoons low-sodium soy sauce
- 1 tablespoon sesame oil

Instructions:
1. In a skillet or wok, heat the sesame oil over medium heat.
2. Add the cooked chicken breast slices and stir-fry for 2-3 minutes until heated through.
3. Add the mixed stir-fry vegetables to the skillet and stir-fry for another 3-4 minutes until tender-crisp.
4. Stir in the cooked brown rice and low-sodium soy sauce.
5. Continue to stir-fry for 2-3 minutes until everything is well combined and heated through.
6. Serve the chicken stir-fry with brown rice and vegetables immediately.

7. Enjoy this customizable and nutrient-dense dinner!

Nutritional Information: (per serving)
Calories: 350 kcal
Protein: 30g, Fat: 10g, Carbohydrates: 35g
Fiber: 6g

Baked Sweet Potato with Black Beans and Salsa

Serving Size: 1 serving

Ingredients:
- 1 medium sweet potato
- 1/2 cup canned black beans, drained and rinsed
- 1/4 cup salsa
- Salt and pepper to taste
- Fresh cilantro for garnish

Instructions:
1. Preheat the oven to 400°F (200°C).
2. Wash the sweet potato thoroughly and pierce it several times with a fork.
3. Place the sweet potato on a baking sheet and bake in the preheated oven for 45-60 minutes, or until tender.
4. Once the sweet potato is cooked, split it open and fluff the flesh with a fork.
5. Top the baked sweet potato with black beans, salsa, salt, and pepper.
6. Garnish with fresh cilantro, if desired.
7. Enjoy this fiber-rich and flavorful meal!

Nutritional Information: (per serving)
Calories: 300 kcal
Protein: 10g, Fat: 1g, Carbohydrates: 65g
Fiber: 12g

Shrimp Scampi over Zoodles

Serving Size: 1 serving

Ingredients:
- 4 oz shrimp, peeled and deveined
- 1 cup zucchini noodles (zoodles)
- 2 cloves garlic, minced
- 1 tablespoon olive oil
- 1 tablespoon lemon juice
- Salt and pepper to taste

Instructions:
1. In a pan over medium heat, warm the olive oil.
2. Add the minced garlic to the skillet and cook it until fragrant, about one to two minutes.
3. When the shrimp are pink and fully cooked, add them to the skillet and sauté them for two to three minutes on each side.
4. Stir in the lemon juice and season with salt and pepper to taste.
5. Add the zucchini noodles to the skillet and toss with the shrimp and garlic mixture.
6. Cook for an additional 2-3 minutes until the zucchini noodles are heated through.
7. Serve the shrimp scampi over zoodles immediately.
8. Enjoy this low-carb and satisfying dinner!

Nutritional Information: (per serving)
Calories: 250 kcal
Protein: 25g, Fat: 10g, Carbohydrates: 10g
Fiber: 3g

One-Pan Chicken with Roasted Vegetables

Serving Size: 1 serving

Ingredients:
- 4 oz chicken breast or thigh, boneless and skinless
- 1 cup mixed vegetables (such as bell peppers, broccoli, and carrots), chopped
- 1 tablespoon olive oil
- Salt and pepper to taste
- Optional: Herbs and spices of your choice

Instructions:
1. Preheat the oven to 400°F (200°C).
2. Place the chicken breast or thigh and mixed vegetables on a baking sheet.
3. Drizzle olive oil over the chicken and vegetables, then season with salt, pepper, and your choice of herbs and spices.
4. Toss everything together to coat evenly.
5. Roast in the preheated oven for 20-25 minutes, or until the chicken is cooked through and the vegetables are tender.
6. Before serving, take it out of the oven and give it some time to rest.
7. Enjoy this effortless and healthy one-pan dinner!

Nutritional Information: (per serving)
Calories: 300 kcal
Protein: 30g, Fat: 12g, Carbohydrates: 15g
Fiber: 5g

Snacks

Apple Slices with Almond Butter

Serving Size: 1 serving

Ingredients:
- 1 medium apple, sliced
- 2 tablespoons almond butter

Instructions:
1. Wash and slice the apple into thin wedges.
2. Spread almond butter on each apple slice.
3. Arrange the apple slices on a plate.
4. Enjoy this simple and healthy snack!

Nutritional Information: (per serving)
Calories: 200 kcal
Protein: 4g, Fat: 10g, Carbohydrates: 25g
Fiber: 5g

Edamame Pods

Serving Size: 1 serving

Ingredients:
- 1 cup edamame pods (frozen or fresh)
- Salt to taste

Instructions:
1. If using frozen edamame pods, thaw them according to package instructions.
2. In a saucepan, bring the water to a boil.
3. Add the edamame pods to the boiling water and cook for 3-5 minutes, or until tender.
4. Drain the edamame pods and sprinkle with salt.
5. Serve immediately as a plant-based protein and fiber-rich snack.

Nutritional Information: (per serving)
Calories: 100 kcal
Protein: 9g, Fat: 3g, Carbohydrates: 8g
Fiber: 4g

Carrot Sticks with Hummus

Serving Size: 1 serving

Ingredients:
- 1 medium carrot, peeled and sliced into sticks
- 2 tablespoons hummus

Instructions:
1. Wash and peel the carrot, then slice it into sticks.
2. Serve the carrot sticks with hummus for dipping.
3. Enjoy this fun and protein-packed snack!

Nutritional Information: (per serving)
- Calories: 150 kcal
- Protein: 5g
- Fat: 8g
- Carbohydrates: 18g
- Fiber: 6g

Greek Yogurt with Berries

Serving Size: 1 serving

Ingredients:
- 1/2 cup Greek yogurt
- 1/4 cup of berries, including blueberries, raspberries, and strawberries

Instructions:
1. Spoon Greek yogurt into a bowl.
2. Top with mixed berries.
3. Stir gently to combine.
4. Enjoy this light and satisfying snack!

Nutritional Information: (per serving)
Calories: 100 kcal
Protein: 12g, Fat: 2g, Carbohydrates: 10g
Fiber: 2g

Air-Fried Chickpeas

Serving Size: 1 serving

Ingredients:
- 1/2 cup cooked chickpeas (garbanzo beans)
- 1 teaspoon olive oil
- Salt and spices of your choice (such as paprika, garlic powder, or cumin)

Instructions:
1. Turn the air fryer on to 400°F, or 200°C.
2. Drain and rinse the cooked chickpeas, then pat them dry with a paper towel.
3. In a bowl, toss the chickpeas with olive oil, salt, and spices until evenly coated.
4. Place the seasoned chickpeas in the basket of the air fryer.
5. Air fry for 15-20 minutes, shaking the basket halfway through, until golden and crispy.
6. Let the chickpeas cool slightly before serving.
7. Enjoy these crunchy and protein-packed snacks!

Nutritional Information: (per serving)
Calories: 150 kcal
Protein: 7g, Fat: 5g, Carbohydrates: 20g
Fiber: 6g

Drinks

Green Tea

Serving Size: 1 cup

Ingredients:
- 1 green tea bag
- 1 cup hot water

Instructions:
1. Fill a cup with the green tea bag.
2. Immerse the tea bag in hot water.
3. Depending on desired strength, steep for three to five minutes.
4. Remove the tea bag and discard.
5. Enjoy this antioxidant-rich beverage!

Nutritional Information: (per serving)
Calories: 0 kcal
Protein: 0g, Fat: 0g, Carbohydrates: 0g
Fiber: 0g

Water with Lemon or Cucumber

Serving Size: 1 glass

Ingredients:
- 1 glass of water
- Slices of lemon or cucumber (optional)

Instructions:
1. Fill a glass with water.
2. Add slices of lemon or cucumber for flavor (optional).
3. Stir gently to infuse the water.
4. Chill in the refrigerator if desired.
5. Enjoy this hydrating and refreshing drink!

Nutritional Information: (per serving)
Calories: 0 kcal
Protein: 0g, Fat: 0g, Carbohydrates: 0g
Fiber: 0g

Unsweetened Herbal Tea

Serving Size: 1 cup

Ingredients:
- 1 herbal tea bag (such as chamomile, peppermint, or ginger)
- 1 cup hot water

Instructions:
1. Place the herbal tea bag in a cup.
2. Over the tea bag, pour some boiling water.
3. Steep for 5-7 minutes, depending on desired strength.
4. Remove the tea bag and discard.
5. Enjoy this flavorful and caffeine-free beverage!

Nutritional Information: (per serving)
Calories: 0 kcal
Protein: 0g, Fat: 0g, Carbohydrates: 0g
Fiber: 0g

Homemade Vegetable Juice

Serving Size: 1 cup

Ingredients:
- Assorted vegetables (such as carrots, spinach, kale, celery)
- Water

Instructions:
1. Wash and chop the vegetables into small pieces.
2. Place the vegetables in a blender.
3. Add water to cover the vegetables.
4. Blend until smooth.
5. Strain the mixture to remove pulp if desired.
6. Serve immediately or chill in the refrigerator.
7. Enjoy this nutrient-dense and hydrating juice!

Nutritional Information: (per serving)
Varies depending on vegetables used

Smoothie with Spinach, Banana, and Water

Serving Size: 1 glass

Ingredients:
- 1 cup fresh spinach leaves
- 1 ripe banana
- 1/2 cup water

Instructions:
1. Place the spinach, banana, and water in a blender.
2. Blend until smooth and creamy.
3. After pouring into a glass, serve right away.
4. Enjoy this low-sugar and filling smoothie!

Nutritional Information: (per serving)
Calories: 100 kcal
Protein: 2g, Fat: 0.5g, Carbohydrates: 25g
Fiber: 3g

Bonus

Fruit Salad with Chia Seeds

Serving Size: 1 bowl

Ingredients:
- Assorted fruits (such as strawberries, blueberries, kiwi, pineapple)
- 1 tablespoon chia seeds

Instructions:
1. Wash and chop the fruits into bite-sized pieces.
2. Place the chopped fruits in a bowl.
3. Sprinkle chia seeds over the fruits.
4. Toss gently to combine.
5. Serve immediately or chill in the refrigerator.
6. Enjoy this light and refreshing fruit salad!

Nutritional Information: (per serving)
Varies depending on fruits used

Hard-boiled Eggs

Serving Size: 2 eggs

Ingredients:
- 2 eggs

Instructions:
1. Put the eggs into a pot and pour water over them.
2. Use high heat to bring the water to a boil.
3. Once boiling, reduce the heat to low and let the eggs simmer for 9-12 minutes, depending on desired doneness.
4. Remove the eggs from the hot water and place them in a bowl of ice water to cool.
5. Once cooled, peel the eggs and serve.
6. Enjoy these portable and protein-rich snacks!

Nutritional Information: (per serving)
Calories: 140 kcal
Protein: 12g, Fat: 10g, Carbohydrates: 1g
Fiber: 0g

Cottage Cheese with Fruit

Serving Size: 1 bowl

Ingredients:
- 1/2 cup cottage cheese
- Assorted fruits (such as peach slices, pineapple chunks, berries)

Instructions:
1. Place the cottage cheese in a bowl.
2. Add the assorted fruits on top of the cottage cheese.
3. Stir gently to combine.
4. Serve immediately.
5. Enjoy this protein and fiber combo snack!

Nutritional Information: (per serving)
Calories: Varies depending on fruits used
Protein: 13g, Fat: 2g

Air-Fried Tofu Scramble with Vegetables

Serving Size: 1 bowl

Ingredients:
- 1/2 cup firm tofu, crumbled
- Assorted vegetables (such as bell peppers, onions, spinach)
- 1 tablespoon olive oil

Instructions:
1. Heat olive oil in a skillet over medium heat.
2. Add the assorted vegetables to the skillet and sauté until tender.
3. Add the crumbled tofu to the skillet and cook until heated through.
4. Sprinkle over some pepper and salt, to taste.
5. Serve immediately.
6. Enjoy this vegan and protein-rich snack!

Nutritional Information: (per serving)
Varies depending on ingredients used

Roasted Pumpkin Seeds

Serving Size: 1/4 cup

Ingredients:
- 1/4 cup pumpkin seeds
- Salt (optional)

Instructions:
1. Set the oven's temperature to 150°C/300°F.
2. Arrange the pumpkin seeds on a baking sheet in a single layer.
3. If desired, top with salt.
4. Roast, tossing periodically, for 20 to 25 minutes in a preheated oven, or until golden brown.
5. When ready to serve, take out of the oven and allow to cool.
6. Savor these crispy, high-protein seeds!

Nutritional Information: (per serving)
Calories: 180 kcal
Protein: 9g, Fat: 15g, Carbohydrates: 4g
Fiber: 2g

14-Day Meal Plan

Week 1

Day 1:
- Breakfast: Greek Yogurt with Berries and Chia Seeds
- Lunch: Tuna Salad with Whole Wheat Crackers
- Dinner: Air-Fried Salmon with Roasted Broccoli
- Snack: Apple Slices with Almond Butter

Day 2:
- Breakfast: Scrambled Eggs with Spinach and Tomatoes
- Lunch: Lentil Soup with Whole Wheat Bread
- Dinner: Chicken Stir-Fry with Brown Rice and Vegetables
- Snack: Edamame Pods

Day 3:
- Breakfast: Oatmeal with Banana and Nuts
- Lunch: Chicken Caesar Salad with Light Dressing
- Dinner: Baked Sweet Potato with Black Beans and Salsa
- Snack: Carrot Sticks with Hummus

Day 4:
- Breakfast: Avocado Toast with Smoked Salmon
- Lunch: Black Bean and Corn Salad with Avocado
- Dinner: Shrimp Scampi over Zoodles
- Snack: Greek Yogurt with Berries

Day 5:
- Breakfast: Smoothie with Spinach, Banana, and Almond Milk
- Lunch: Leftover Grilled Chicken or Fish with Roasted Vegetables
- Dinner: One-Pan Chicken with Roasted Vegetables
- Snack: Air-Fried Chickpeas

Day 6:
- Breakfast: Apple Slices with Almond Butter
- Lunch: Tuna Salad with Whole Wheat Crackers
- Dinner: Air-Fried Salmon with Roasted Broccoli
- Snack: Edamame Pods

Day 7:
- Breakfast: Scrambled Eggs with Spinach and Tomatoes
- Lunch: Lentil Soup with Whole Wheat Bread
- Dinner: Chicken Stir-Fry with Brown Rice and Vegetables
- Snack: Cottage Cheese with Fruit

Week 2

Day 8:
- Breakfast: Oatmeal with Banana and Nuts
- Lunch: Chicken Caesar Salad with Light Dressing
- Dinner: Baked Sweet Potato with Black Beans and Salsa
- Snack: Carrot Sticks with Hummus

Day 9:
- Breakfast: Avocado Toast with Smoked Salmon
- Lunch: Black Bean and Corn Salad with Avocado
- Dinner: Shrimp Scampi over Zoodles
- Snack: Greek Yogurt with Berries

Day 10:
- Breakfast: Smoothie with Spinach, Banana, and Almond Milk
- Lunch: Leftover Grilled Chicken or Fish with Roasted Vegetables
- Dinner: One-Pan Chicken with Roasted Vegetables
- Snack: Air-Fried Chickpeas

Day 11:
- Breakfast: Greek Yogurt with Berries and Chia
Seeds
- Lunch: Tuna Salad with Whole Wheat Crackers
- Dinner: Air-Fried Salmon with Roasted Broccoli
- Snack: Apple Slices with Almond Butter

Day 12:
- Breakfast: Scrambled Eggs with Spinach and
Tomatoes
- Lunch: Lentil Soup with Whole Wheat Bread
- Dinner: Chicken Stir-Fry with Brown Rice and
Vegetables
- Snack: Edamame Pods

Day 13:
- Breakfast: Oatmeal with Banana and Nuts
- Lunch: Chicken Caesar Salad with Light Dressing
- Dinner: Baked Sweet Potato with Black Beans and
Salsa
- Snack: Carrot Sticks with Hummus

Day 14:
- Breakfast: Avocado Toast with Smoked Salmon
- Lunch: Black Bean and Corn Salad with Avocado
- Dinner: Shrimp Scampi over Zoodles
- Snack: Greek Yogurt with Berries

CONCLUSION

As we come to the end of our adventure through the "Fatty Liver Diet Cookbook for Seniors 2024," I would like to express my sincere appreciation to each and every one of you for starting this life-changing journey. We've looked at scrumptious, nutrient-dense dishes on these pages that are especially suited to seniors who are living with fatty liver disease. As we say goodbye to these gastronomic explorations, keep in mind that wellbeing and health are continual journeys rather than destination. We are motivated to keep offering helpful tools for your wellbeing by your commitment to adopting healthy eating habits and your support in doing so.

I hope you discover new life and happiness in feeding your body and spirit as you implement these recipes into your everyday routine. I cordially encourage you to rate and review this book so that others might benefit from your ideas and experiences. Your suggestions not only help us become better, but they also inspire other seniors to start their own paths to improved health. We appreciate you sharing your health journey with us. Let's work together to continue giving everyone who seeks it the gift of excellent health and a clean lifestyle.